The Voyage

The Voyage

[A Play]

J. Lea Koretsky

REGENT PRESS
Berkeley, California

ISBN 13: 978-1-58790-261-1
ISBN 10: 1-58790-261-3
Library of Congress Catalog Number: 2103955550

Manufactured in the U.S.A.
REGENT PRESS
Berkeley, California
www.regentpress.net
regentpress@mindspring.com

ACT 1

Scene 1

(In a graveyard wth grey stone patio and garden near Antartica.)

PHYSICIAN :

My work may come before I know the wit
Must be for all reserved a fright obscure
Benign or tempered claim doth spaeke a swift
Departure forth a cruel stiff knife to lure,
Who knows what fate in every breath awaits
If penalty or cure refrains its sap
Breaks skin while sewn treacherous blood sates
The whims of love can hope to purge the knap,
In search of portals beast to find a door
Who goes through mist is transform stellar mate
Erudite change that leaves no wound nor fore
To fester deep aggregate misery late,
The years bestow in life desirous fate
Who finds all strengths blessings sung to loved jade.
I can neither say bed or grace well suits
Dedication brings wings in years to stay
A keeper one may have if trove fruits
Treasured rejoice of kind relief make way,
As I save lives in honest practice sums
As long as one imparts no mind of God
He joins in quest that they and he are one
In truth suffers as they heal limb from shod,
Daylight with stars fading dispel nairy

The Voyage

I chase the deaths of life into remote
Although I've come upon wretched few fairy
Bandaged, lean-to's, herbal regrets devote,
The travel ship doctor must mast for winds
To where sunlight detects Morte's parting sins.

ACT 1

Scene 2

(In an enclosed garden in Victoria, South Africa.)

WIFE :

If only life should pledge an oath for two
Emotions mock the rarest food to choose
Pastures embrace a devious miscue
Tender visions describe letters with Muse,
Had I a thousand just like him to yearn
A yard complete in each girl's heart would snare
Medicinal pleasures might surely burn
When lights turned low give most of bare,
The world played would situate its stock
Whisper tidings adjourned in liens of bide
A bride's true blush cavort with earnest pluck
That mercy may gain while charters pride,
In far seeking matters the sought redeems
Method for method keeps all truth esteems.

SON :

The wife's prayers answer soothing through storm
Companion dear who walks the clock assist
Prevails when Sleep governs the dark of morn
When naught reduce the will dispelled of rift,
In her finest hour her kiss relieves
Skillful arbitration supports a guileless aim
A cleanly home enjoys the bake achieves

The herb garden grows tall in patient rain,
Partnership requires steady discourse for health
Absence apart wanders a merry glance
At sea twenty and ten sever men's stealth
His soul flounders alone in doubtful stance,
Cleopatra created coffins to house
The light from ship on ocean's Furies douse.
Shibboleth subdued a new world by sword
Slowness treating village of bite ailments
Even false entreaty prisons by lured
To which pestilence condemns by splints,
He wrote his wife asking she forgive him
All life deterred spirits after that siege
He lay subtract in gauze to cancel tin
His mind and mood did threat to snap aggrieve,
Each ship could plan afar to lands abroad
To wilderness to hunt in brush for cures
With strong material cloth were held prompt stored
Sorrows plainly perceived throughout endures,
Afraid and lost imbued by feverish fear
Hoping to be restored in limb past leer.

SON'S SON :

Concubines and patriarchs both may flee
Escape portal image in mist of beast
Slither or shoot arrows of flint melee
Deduce by hour the caged coquet to cease,
At home worry consumes all pride swiftly
Enjoins sorry laments in twisted rank
Covets comfort secure for late carry
Mischief folly beckons rascal ill prank,
About the house we seek a mask to find

Borrow vitals as one might hunt a prey
Induce common complaint to make its kind
Subdue the sense that years befit a pay,
Arise at night moonlight a fetching stay
No ship at dock during abated weak quay.

Friend, a Physician :

Your son is son of mine no less cousin
If he has none the breath of husband sole
He has often a head and heart dozen
Mending ruthless fine stings about the foal,
A worst tender complicated morsel
Of whose very young soul doth make a look
Only a once forget of face the bell
Should one foresee the like of most mistook,
Had I acquired of all the house a shame
I know I may resound my play release
For I alone describe your face in fame
Without the maze of hurt proclaim the feast,
Of all pardons, age sins that might agree
Damned right are we to wed our fates unseen.
I have often wandered afar of you
To bless that which is blessed by none avail
The scars I bear are last a moor for rue
The pains I rake I keep at dearth a rail,
As chimes of lads gone pace in hearts to hell
Heaven's closer than acrimonial grace
Every sunlight I find nearer to quell
Distance bemused entwined of our mistake,
I hold you dear by day lest I awake
Foolish a trap that holds my foot in place
If he rethinks himself a doctor's sake

So I do tend your cares with fond disgrace,
For you I have no home apart of life
You shine as none but truest hopes which knife.

Wife :

I've told myself chancery lies bed with him
His sweet goodbye tender blue waves
Of rising spheres liven on polar wren
Affix sorrow isles remarks to stave,
I can no more subscribe meanest entreaties
Nor queer of nets be fetched by helm's tears
Acquiesce oblivion miscast as enemies
Or starve my cries an acrobat of steers,
Try not to leave fevered gasping actor
For I shall keep mercy slaking content
If you insist I walk a path to war
Knowing full well you are my better rent,
Improper circumstance induces clear trace
Duty I am forsworn to dearest lace.
Some day ironic tax shall prod its bud
And I may find I lack sunny bestow
Discovery unkind embarrass mud
If not outright assume a puzzling blow,
Enigma's signs alight with craft most pique
Enjoyed allure a fortune found to bait
While joy like Time doth grant all pleas bespake
Predawn with dark revile may spend the gate,
Could I assure allays a bow complete
Inform you each of house and fortune blessed
I could soon leave senses before replete
And scorn myself a femme unfaith distressed,
But damned I'm not under the stars zenith

My youth complicated by lonely wreath.

Friend :

Now come, let's find ourselves secluded from yore
That I may ask of you all fond designs
Grandson and son encroach upon the lore
Seeking least mirth or ridicule's blue wine,
Retort offends mirror it cannot see
Recalls impolite mire for jest occur
Goodness no one will reap for years of tea
Censure a trickster's yarn love's tears to blur,
I know my charms may be your better fortune
That secrecy doth bolt a door of truth
But now we are of age where schemes stay ruin
My hands implore of you be kinder soothe,
Inspire my age with purities enchant
Boldly pursue me now without recant.

Secretary :

(Enters from right wing, reading paper.)

My lord sends word danger appeared at britch
About the stern engrossed a wraith sanguine
The mast poles swung into a gale pitch
The poor ice light gave heaving winch a blind,
Limitation quarantined wit for loss
Determined philanthropy narcotic
A sedative good choice orthodox
Orphan misgivings dear to life's comic,
Despite lax attitudes polarity
Mania, panic, offense and infection

The crew has posed no insincere malty
Islands redeemed they shipped smarten,
Self-deception hastens collusion free
Does bind eradicate intention see.
Knots more delicate wind long streams assured
Flounder high seas in eerie echoes last
Destruct human laid plans of every fleur
Quagmire deceit congealed designs cast,
A few more years I may accrue this debt
Obliged by late telescript to lend subscribe
Ornary men conjure the worst roulette
Until drunken despise their weakest tide,
Could I but tell who gives the day its ditty
Or plaits straddle the horse his jump high fence
Retreat we might in vans psychology
Too far aspire random or ration one's rents,
Dearest, forgive my vain disputes outwit
Each injunction and contention befit.

WIFE :

(Goes over to secretary.)

Of where did you obtain that note in scrawl
How oft' has it been read about the wharf
Why was I not informed at once landfall
While all forsook did plunge my love false morph,
How can I tend to love if I mislearn
That brief a chart went wrong at sea rely
If bell did warn of ice and waves fang churn
Fallow fairly spun wheel to knee decry,
Who wants me shamed farthest farewell unknown
Must I far-sight reveal fallible falcon

I may have seen eyebright the tempt a home
Why must I wait the heart's stolen defection,
That years astern proclaim no advantage
Like hoary thieves we wait revoke visage.

SON'S SON :

(Off to side.)

Does she not see that all the world rejects
Her pleas for carriage brimmed divulge the store
E'en Dad retorts it's naught a quest deflects
Scylla may decimate arrows deplore,
Ransack the flour and delegate decency
Shower fond deficit in laps lunar
Her husband presumed true as nobility
His skint hardly skewered trona sooner,
Woman's anger has none steadfast to be
Twenty short years has she to grieve his leave
A mariner is pact seasons galley
Astute to apostle purpose rack undeceive,
His love for her never not dreams forgot
A tight held leash relieves the troth faucet.

WIFE :

(Overhearing him, talks to Secretary.)

To what ailment ought I address myself
Fallacy is fanatic fan opposed extent
I gave my surgeon gloves away for kelp
Lament this skill an altruist portent,
I knew my life as well to be futile

A hapless sting disposed was lost in strings
Traded milepost for Faust to gain domicile
For all that vigilance insures it brings,
There are rich sins worthy of parole's dance
Scowl or laugh a foal forgives its shoal
My doctor blessed, it is his son love's lance
Ampoule directed aim describes control,
Opium for Nefertiti
Mystic myrtle mutilate neat charity.

SON :

The son doth mend the broken heart astray
Doth make its turn a brief behold release
As gods will sun and moon the best betray
Only surmount a play covets bane's lease,
The doctor wise may find privy dispute
All words cannot their fans govern afar
For what is love but small matters refute
Or slate that which may stake destined man's par,
I give the chill knowledgeable instinct
The sum of cause relives stymied fastice
Revels descript of pleasure bound intrigue
Kind knife the cord is drawn as found justice,
She walks among summer flowers wilted
He lives despite no grace portend jilted.
What must I say to wreak no havoc claim
The way surmise its craft beguiles lessen
The masts release with speed capture disdain
If life renews with love in haste petition,
Sorrow keeps few mortal jealous sentence
It saves nor earns a pensioner's disquiet
Revolves its gaze upon lustrous sentience

Until tiresome swain relieves his fight,
Analytic mendacity oppose
Briefer stillborn goodwill deters its chase
Favorite fear becomes the swill's dispose
When fancy free employs a dunned mistake,
Hold close that which one ought more sense let go
To grieve the fates that shorn the minor oath.

Wife :

(Mother of Son.)

I have allowed my life to find you true
My most granted fortune Salish sculpture
Are we contained at home by will or clue
Endure of stage the winds salty rapture,
You heard your father's wise reply demands
Perhaps more than ten years at sea repent
Thus mere thirty long suns I may commend
Stave off lyric malfeasance sage entrant,
You are alone my soul for waking age
Insights are host among reminders matched
Doctor yourself humanity's birdcage
Asylum the tender lives who must be fetched,
I take your hand in solemn grasp to guide
Findings scholar mantic diptych confide.

Son :

How right you were to urge early divorce
A hundred smite calamities arose
Ketosis, anxiety, heretic course
Sinister hysteria endorsed saros,

Despicable cravings bulimic slice
Became engaged sacrifice bled practice
If run I did, my soaring hope lay diced
Like inflammation elliptic axis,
My contestant heir son argues the night
He steals by day fetching die-cast tidings
He was too young to learn his mother's blight
Or make his education of poised innings,
But he is Life for whom I am conceived
Your oft' blessings in turn grant him believed.

Wife :

Imprecise acts woven into thin veils
Are oft' merry deceit reviled imposter
We are like one ripple intuit through gales
Always the other the repairer mirror,
Should loves be found by meager fault confess
If you or I lose track paths shall establish
Madness directs the mind over regress
Disloyalties create the wind that loops enmesh,
Just so, collapse may warrant swift denial
Outwit prudish beliefs from grim barrage
Loosen a home with leave imperils labile
Its douche a garish yellow sabotage,
Despondence neutralized to reversal
Cockerel leanings pose floral rehearsal.

Son :

How cynical your wit about Hazel
She means no harm nor requital killjoy
After all spoons, she is my son's gavel

Marital remittal requires assured ploy,
You liked her once when Dad was home a year
He said she infected him with warm aim
That she with me completed an epicure
Dark curls and laughing stride forgave acclaim,
With child she grew taciturn and craving
Complaints of brooding diminished her love
Possessively envious of womb she knew no haven
At William's birth she shunned the babe behove,
It was the first I spied defeat of kin
Tragedy erred on quilts tending to fin.
Disenfranchised one gets nowhere but slain
Beckons with grace livened of staid remorse
Discerned failure an unholy rain
A cheese refrain of glory departed course,
Winter's cheap draft a veritable remain
Clandestined redress barometer graveyard
Method by hills crimson peonies gain
Although the breeze cancels finer reward,
I have answered the call of youth aware
As plaid a marsh may wear honest distill
Throughout the brim my cup is filled of fare
Knowest thine eyes every keen branch is ill,
You have my heart and all its buds fulfilled
Treasure and scope that brave enfolds in tills.

Wife :

Father your gains that you may seed your race
I'm told the blessed account the years are stored
Heaven's foothold revised for earnest place
The wheels of time beget regrets implored,
So much have we to darn our staid response

Follies are yet kindled unkind despair
I gave my breast notions of love constants
Too soon ambiguity began its dare,
Your flesh travels afar for terror demise
Kindred species bespeak single picture
One peninsula bleak might crease a rise
If speed gives not a sum of cured fixture,
Described to me are but a moment's notice
Of health and squalor impertinent mortise.

SON'S SON :

You two entwine to make a bank of vows
Religious rigor at a husband's table
Deferred caress cannot relieve your rows
For Faith assures proper livery stable,
I heard you speak of descent clear of mine
You Ma'am did chase your fledgling bride from home
No shame show you toward surname nor twine
You seek the yard as one may fetch a bone,
Twice week the man doth touch your fleeing skirts
His kiss must gleam its stark betrayal to sea
I won't wonder when he returns whose mirth
We must retort to ease stolen hours nee,
Why fell the grass with displeasing candor
If married to solitaire you gave ardor.

FRIEND :

(Stepping onto the patio having slept off a draught.)

Who speaks? Unkindly lad you vow to be
Straight off the bench in cut and lout pant cut

A reconnoiter cap atop a whiskey
You'd best train late in nurse sponge bitternut,
Cuckoo crooner, delirium or crutch crick
Insults to your grand lair you may astride
Take sauce elsewhere the damp will not afflict
Apology restrict your gambol ride,
You think tokens of insincere redact
Stupors vanquished for him detained at sea
We are not for wanton charms sense lacked
Nor caps stagger like hens to prey rea,
Were you younger I'd slap your knees with whip
Cull your impulse of sly condemned quip.

SON :

(Spoken to mother's friend.)

The best of life is yet to come to terms
That you may try affect disgrace with words
Lofty spellbound simulates particular firms
Decide a plan merits often its herds,
With whom you live depends on struck ill girds
Rhetoric displacement retrograde still
Misdeeds carnivore relation heard
Decades of masquerade produce will,
Astral astounds green wreaths of aspiring
Extraterrestrial facsimile
Endeavored reach for platitudes fowling
Bourne curiosity decreed astronomy,
The further you assert to ascend to art
You leave behind the choice undoing apart.

ACT 2

Scene 1

(On an isle off Tasmania.)

PHYSICIAN :

Though winds that blow of salty air dismay
The men are safe within their coastal hut
Wild boars were shot by guns fired relay
Slattern fierce rains abated windows shut,
About marine skiver the hold did sink
A slash of might it took to slide a rise
Sleepless torment skewed slag's sane brink
Defiled skid ways skittish did spring alight,
Cautious became telltale wind spout adjourn
Weather voyagers sent to gale outposts
To verify height speed of waves nocturne
Splatter extremes hurled far in typhoon soaks,
Mutiny harsh wave crashers emancipated
Trenches built deep in host rock strata equated.
Daybreak wolf packs arranged on hills did strike
Ghastly damage to homes was done intrude
Horrified range like limbs bullets might
Deviate hymns inquired service collude,
We blundered on in toils confusing uproar
Wavered for obstruction against the ground
All hands tackled limits of hoisted vigor
Churlish babble disarmed spoilage resound,
Neap tide great plates of ice all blue did slide
Across the straits Afrjca's droll did pale

Currents awash deafened erratic hide
Befell sluggish deluge attained in ail,
For this I ventured seas to acquiesce
Giving suture, brandy, consoling relapse.
Who is to say instructs uncover hormones
That once we land allures exert a fine
Fleeting fatigue in dead of heat forgone
Ravings tarnish like sparse rebuffs are sign
Of mindless eyes that weep cerise react
Dislocations of every sort were swelled
Desolate wails sacrificed ramp distract
Endurance brief digressed with vim compelled,
Alone I leaned on crutch of care perform
Reject alarmed spirographic chart
Disposition augment battle mend form
Squinting gazes required skilled remark,
Let jinx think not a hyperbole be
Occult menace the bower almonry.

Female Nurse :

(In her twenties, islander, blond Australian.)

In truth I was aware of Wife's affairs
Because he imbued strident rung like the son
By kidnap he should decry his sore repairs
Revoked fidelity undone,
Why fantasy conjures its cradle-song
Perforates blush indelible gambit
Blemish stricken purchase with banished wrong
I stay close by in hopes he needs sedate,
Waters of this kindly fashion stir trapped
Epidemic cramped muscle wounds confer

Ramble about the edge of tent is strapped
While thought carries only image caper,
Brown blood distinguished gush did surge
Cuckold mimicry on sphymograph purge.
Daily island people are fed diet
Mash soup to rise impugned ill scheme
Lean bodies examined for famine's riot
Gladiators dictatorship unseen,
Worsted tears spurt without plowman's garden
Grapery thorns punish instigators
Too few penitent revive to barter
Inedible concourse doth map factors,
Although the veranda is tangible
And cataracts a trait lost sight profane
Dandy creates his bloom invincible
For fate rustic mire mends by cocaine,
We wait for day to pronounce toil its end
Before we eat, sacrifice repent mend.

Physician:

(Writes to Son.)

Wish Mother well, tell her I pray the stars
Shall fix my life that I may come home soon
Boathouse, garden, crop farms, grapery, pars
Are built sturdy withstand frothy high moon,
Gave alms and bed linen with wash basins
Motionless mourn threatens our station
Unadorned dress and finer fabric evasion
To keep away insects from lit occasion,
Your son must have complete his health studies
Taken post doctorate in front of law

The Voyage

On two sail ships letters he wrote, muddied
Sanctions for ship permit father son slaw,
Hoist, tackle, crank, dredge, ramp the masts give way
Heave-ho low tide the mud doth churn mainstay.
Shabby desire may not sedate mistrust
Nor love move oars passionate gain revive
Candor where good policy has long fussed
Creates both surge and blush rejoice alive,
Finder's keeper may not be poor a choice
If new win's child likeable interest
Have you relentless pursuit in chaste voice
Many obscured females shall entwine tress,
Of course the matters of heart come first in maze
Graces are encountered in life when senses lose
That most precious discerns the least of daze
Mortems reduce for aims of fallen rues,
Here at my side my nurse employs assist
Long days punish hourly fractures remiss.
By vise or will I keep my life display
Sixty interns may rope the boats on ice
We place our lives on cliffs conjured stay
For fear we lose the life of he with vice,
Among stilled breath must he enjoy relief
All told mauve fidelity walks apart
Reality soon fools bungled disease
Enjoins cashier that lies betrayed its guard,
Desire permits no fellatio to rob
Instinct bereft doth sing its keeper's praise
That which abides goodbye of dock a mob
Pretends sole cloughs are swept in rainy days,
I shall return to hear you speak your keen
Capable wit adhered by charming mean.

INTERN 1 :

(To Nurse.)

Does he yet know howling destroys its porch
Locates the point finite redact of muse
One starts the bridge to find the sky a gorge
Where men lost foot and fell in kind review,
Suture, bandage, cure spleen, reduce venom
Remark revive, tent air, alleviate
Displace burdened pressure in bloods sternum
Cerebral hemorrhage invites deviate,
Absorbs agnostic allopathy heal
Alcoholic delusion nature stems
Aldosterone sitologies reveal
Assure the cutting grafts of iced periblems,
I turn to you to loosen binds of cloth
Checkmate tourniquet needless gushing clot.

INTERN 2 :

(To both.)

Motto travel is die if you must live
Know self better than betrayal's keeper
Wail over misbegotten vindictive
Poultice rashes with clogged foxglove reaper,
Enlist tranquil caudex resolve appendix
Digestive drink morphine extractive
Warm oil in ears cartilage anthelix
Sweet peony illusions derivative,
I have treated tropics poetics matchbox
Struggled against sermon for enlighten

Watched clock hands twirling spin heady aloft
Revitalize with fluids deplanked revision,
Sturdy as hope heavenly stairs alight
The closed door returns to earth the man from flight.

Nurse :

Morbid discuss renews fondest fable
A shriek won't harm the lads who teach the youth
If bells re-ring to gather public stable
Rushes lilac imbed lanterns with ruth,
The stile pretense weans bland fair remorse
Ancient density accepts Nordic stonehenge
As though famed fright reviled in dismal gore
Charity blest on silver wings dawn tinged,
Lofty peril arisen of wastes below
Ignores laments when haste codifies sense
Able hands describe marshy convent furrow
Mixture weakness candid lifetime till rense,
Black knots, fish strewn, life flies amidst the mists
Lines drawn, nets pulled, choirs chant despair enlists.

Physician :

(Joins her, asks them to leave.)

Sunset recounts numerous tales of brave
Likewise upon return I shall see dusk
In rows order produces flowers that rave
Sorrowful night when ballerinas scythe husk,
Bit drunk I be if west befalls east skies
Craving passion to redeem patience swift
I'd care whether the moon in gold rises

Or plummets like a plum engorged of gift,
Dear Renee, let's dance til dawn quivers showers
Of rain and pink bowers a host released
Be mine careless of weeping tender hours
Until you lose all sense of staid beliefs,
I know that you adorn yourself for me
My keenest eye esteems your goodness keep.

NURSE:

I will neither enlist myself a fool
Nor ask after sudden alteration find
You are my dearest friend of which I'm tool
I can no more cause grief than read your mind,
Had fancy struck you and dine left you marred
Were I honest appraise of divine intent
Would you while we are free love me as far
Diminished worth I'd happily pretend,
Yet you are strong in moral dignities
I ought no more to aid your stormy aims
Setting both paths to wreak wrestling enmities
Ashore poorly equipped delays poor fames,
Adore I must so handsome intellect
Creature in me woes inheritor picked.

PHYSICIAN :

(Takes her in his arms and kisses her.)

Lights out.

ACT 2

Scene 2

Physician :

(Alone in garden.)

My life was quenched by easy seduction
On fire my being swiftly purchased align
I wept within to know I found reduction
A lie released I took desire's design,
I said my vows like one possessed by right
Relief so pained I bound a husband's collar
Returned a joy ensemble skiff afterlife
Sailed the shroff to trim recuperator,
Anemic I was for days after profess
Hypnotic dreams on continental drifts
Laughter lavish fretting I did repress
Episodic febrific ache in chaotic grifts,
Enchanted to discover myself delirious
Benefactor actor I submitted psoas.
Remitted on pillowslip Homeric weal
A saccharin sequel endowed reckless
I slant tiller to her thighbone ordeal
Tinsel offered greedy puck selfless,
Errands opiate turgid turmoil trance
Opulence an ordinance web privet
Grievous mirage that has every nuance
Libelous randy which brims its caveat,
Luminous inviolate leave me not bereft
Shore me incorporate I be not fleeced

Grant me a stay should I disgrace accept
Subjugate incurable discontent crease,
If permutable melancholy inscapes
Impractical advance tragic escapes.
I thought amid voluble chatter
With shirt half on I ran to operate
Syrupy err cloying credit platter
Sanity a whip did rejuvenate,
Despite intent to find arteriole
Beneficial slaughter gaudy strumpet
Forgave emotion's outpouring pistoile
I stood so close in surgery to covet,
Unforeseen bronchial release gave toil
Syringe to Keloid scar did turn ascend
Beneath supple scalpel oppose looked spoil
Tedium reimbursed artery descend,
Triage must there baffled fix formation
For mort not be autumn's cancelation.
Through dedicated altruistic accord
I've searched my soul for didactic repent
Scholared afar morbid deceit deplored
Such will conveys mutagenic relent,
Descript elbow yields affection far
Provocation lacking perverse aggress
Doth find its whim castrate casual star
Each tenderness sober recants confess,
Lease me to love's altar converse clever
Deceiver elicits luminous tonus
Dour rebuttal seeks swab endeavor
Victor sympathy undermines onus,
What shall my wife display for nameless purse
True love chalice my lips adore her first.
Taxis like sharks lit roofs through parking streets

The Voyage

Ought I to bless a hearse to cleave her severed
We have married long and find tolerance meets
All definition sums express forever,
Envy is not her suit nor fool's duress
If youth describes even myopic partisan
Elation of triangulation rejects
Pedestal vestiges pertain artisan,
Self-denial while not prescribed bestows
Vintage dotage that disparages facile
Transcends ravish above lenient foes
Doctors systemic chaos in binge servile,
If playing cards wins fortune astute prayer
Could artichokes bring summation despair?
August dismantles her flighty obsess
From summers breeze the haste concludes a kiss
Rectified offerings surrender madcap possess
Winter is dressed in consummate bliss,
Volleys account for sinned wagers randy
Dubious bribery tangos its horse
A cart pulled by reclusive sweet brandy
Defines all acts a crystalline source,
Despite provincial credential I abhor
Soporific dismay that scrolls backwards
That takes sad Assumption spices ignore
Reduces moral blindness to steep fjords,
Were confession better suited to psalms
Could doves depart under prudent qualms?
Too excessive I belabor aflame
Moonbeams become ventured arduous witness
Carnage arousal supplies queer defame
I have nothing to be ashamed fitness,
Sanctions described must be conceit fancy
Maniacal jealousy claim, remote notion

Travesty trucks fetish bewitching piquancy
Nor liked delivery absent devotion,
Fascination may cultivate dual
Spigot strengthen miserly heaven reap
Orchard the balmy confiscate fuel
Advise impulse its clairvoyant leap,
Undoing truth becomes foresight's clue
Recall wonder produces purveyor's view.

ILLUSION :

(Female who resembles Wife enters.)

You must not blame this romantic hunger
For Life seeks neither franchise nor cause
That which has housed your hopes decries asunder
Marriage most blessed borrows a suitor's pause,
Capricious burglary like rancor
Mischievous hereditist hides result
Ransacking hind myopia negator
Stolen your love betraying grim insult,
Comprehends landscape heroism hindered
Has liberated thief of sands likeness
Merciless mercenary pecan wintered
Overripe owns an overdue ellipsis,
You can't have learned by Fate's denials
Sate senses abort favored reprisals.
Feeble febrile anchor keeps hard the dock
Leaves no undertaking a false promise
It plays on edges of knowledge safe mock
Falters kindly in roseate remiss,
I have awaited your sense contrived imbued
Looked for enjoyment ailed to state my words

Watched you toil in depths more wretched stoop
Contained deplore of you abased by lures,
It's worth the hand you take does keep your trust
Far best that love forgives your spoilt wept
Too brief is love and life snowblink combust
Too few remarks which speed destined maps swept,
If you remain you may achieve folly
Entwined are they your love rides bigamy.

Physician :

I've heard this soliloquy once before
When I tested for Army on Andaman
The fact I took to heart gave me bolt sore
I knew certain the paved road lay unplanned,
Marital evidence shows no favor
I am possessed of love in every way
Constance partakes of only food savor
In sleep she cries my name in pray's repay,
I see you wish the best to have decreed
I too allow the heart to bear its crush
Acknowledge none, my wife solely I reed
She lacks fickle yearning of trickster's blush,
When fate declares me free she shall comfort
Her winged suture shall repair Love's chariot.

ACT 3

(Laughter backstage; wife and friend emerge.)

WIFE :

Come here, let me straighten and knot your tie
Be a good boy, take your briefcase by train
Wipe off my berry scone with this nice rye
Give me a hug, here's a chocolate jane.

(Friend leaves.)

SON'S SON :

How many guests are deemed last guests enough
Where one must go for life's living beliefs
To whom must one appeal requisite cuff
Presume candor conveys vulgar relief?
Shall you merrily prance when he returns?

WIFE :

I pray don't be hasty in fault finding
I am cherished to him as he to me
Florid capture is not always kindly
Never have I taken leaving release
Affection wears its ring for all to see.

SON'S SON :

Aye, unholy matrimony concedes

Where even lusty bigotry gives spite
When your husband walks through that door who sees?
Many may be too few to view with right,
Shall you alight then to perjure duty?

WIFE :

What does his letter say about voyage?

SON'S SON :

Six months face time to wean your lover gone.

WIFE :

It may surprise your coop to learn your blood
I have no despicable unremitted wrong
My virtue mislaid does acquaint the rood
Your foul language beseeches unaware song.

SON'S SON :

The partisan environment wearies you
Seasonable sequel reshuffles insurrect
You a lusty petticoat ought flee all rue
Appease your haughty coax canon sect.

WIFE :

My tutor lies hankering to my bosom
Pity shall not inveigh the courier ship
A brush with shabby cultivations come
Steering vandal and thunder obey grip.

Son's son :

Uncivilized Psyche, tyranny's tart
Inhabits indulgent forays slumber
Boorish rapture gone in windless scarce start
Precipitous bondage that lies asunder.

Wife :

I am desired once offered his protege
Neglect you speak incorrect sums the bait
Slave sentiment across vast boundless fey
Attentions smitten by intimate late.

Son's son :

I defer despised weakness that you perish
Acute misery exceeds rivaled rook
A crooked calculated stunt, frugal garish
If thunderous stealth suggests to bait one's hook,
Suspend suspicion deny treachery
Be unlooked for, thrive as best one may
Flounder mackerel that flies clumsy
Trowel extent should cellar try relay,
I bid to show the stump his social class
Gentry disagreeable token status.

Wife :

If he wanders I can't hold my breath
Hours sustain by spent treasure routine
Stalemate from eternal calendar wreath
Bury summits in mausoleums preen,

Attend unbearable monotony
Catapult heady jigger of love
Stingy wastrel of possessive fatigue
Idle leisure produced your excess blood,
Authentic rig debilitating squall
Nothing to do with humiliation
Vaccine against lachrymose pall
Can be not blessed in atypical creation,
Impartial immunity protest stung reliance
For thrilled bloom did grow in surfeit defiance.

SON'S SON :

Does my father know your sharp dismal claim
That he surfeit disposed has no calling
Unsavory jaundice deter by blame
Unabashed joy incurable dallying,
Who are we to you but hid in measure
Contrite or fleet does life suggest pasture?

WIFE :

Although Man may say love is impeached
This is no vaccine against impotency
Immunities surrender groves achieved
Brilliant daylight to stars chronology,
For when the mocking dove sings out of tune
The orb abundance shines fresh ally
Hearsay resents its vacate lot resume
While aloof joined unravels retreat galley,
Here crouched we are until at last we die
Dissent repelled one's honor defrayed wine
Advantage fresh that mitigates desirous cry

Dispels symbolism torrential design,
Who shows the hand of love forgot its grace
Steeps discordance beneath propriety's face?

(She leaves.)

SON'S SON :

Like buds of May your breath makes me seem free
Construe a world that shall hold us unmarred
Be transparent always decor boast serene
Attend cheerless disease by combined starred,
Love you complete until senses are lost
Tell me again you are barren ill-fated
Cancel hours demise what you sought
Briefest wonders a show obey more sated,
I lack no hint of your dim elations
Nor fight thunder approximate vandal
Unkind gesture doth play the door's relations
Borrow unsightly penchant dormant scandal,
Had heaven to imbibe a toxic slate
Be fed the breast of grief its haughty gate.
Where would I stand amused except to bite
Relation is queerly joined far in sieve
The moments worthy a journey respite
While sin is purged exact mislaid reprieve,
Who gains that which is shunned for love's depart
Or quests begot are felled as might connives
Who grants the pony his station pulled cart
Takes youth astray to winch a lad revives,
Were I a sail to find winds ashore fresh
Compass my way to isles forlorn on ice
Had I to ask what lies about the stress

And walk on stratified toppled crevice,
I would aloof entwine my orb to see
Fated abundance modify my reed.
What shall I greet my grandfather's return
Say his son knows less than the world blessed
Adorn his miles in recompense astern
Opiate revision seeks naught distressed?
Will I regain from sight this rude aggress
Display disenfranchised imitate stave
Conquer breath as one who equates profess
Bitter empiric dreams which leave no grave,
Discern neither feud nor cautious umbrage
Leave lit the blue candle in sight of call
Behind basin turn down music storm-bridge
Regress my thought to small images forestall,
I shall greet him kindly most treasured friend
Who with every breath guides me to mend.

ACT 4

(On an island dock having just de-planked; waiting to go to Tasmania.)

PHYSICIAN :

The snow relentlessly does fall on land
Storm's petty churlish scape covers its grades
Who but for whim requires high waves on sand
Mighty coveted cloaking doth sneak parades,
If west is east and east lies south governed
When this little dinghy flies north to reel
Feint pulse Virtue with deity shall mourn
Bereft of light afar the bird its keel,
Shoulder dark wind harnessed in mollusk turn
Billowy masts by night withdrawn unfurled
The brave on deck shall whip the wheel astern
Find hull and rudder sloshed and rain hail curled,
The fix is killed with engines loud recoiled
The crops they carry not yet undisturbed spoiled.
Afar the waves churning above the din
The lens master has spied a prowling boat
Captured by ropes the ocean brings the fin
Hollering the wind unleashes planks soaked,
I fear we might jump ship in this windy gale
The host set sail four days ago is lost
The wake and pitch describe the meanest rail
All ties to timber swung wide of cross,
Intends to savagely dent quay in chalk
Stillborn a hunt-bound ship to ice ghostlike
Break clavicle wrench sock above the lock

Emit bench worth demons in mists down pike,
If ship hull cracks apart the deck will jeer
Putty saves only when the wood can hear.

Intern 3 :

There's sure to be a monster down below
Swaggers left then right a fist might adjourn
Pulls up heavy the sides to breathe a blow
Puts back to bed a sigh of courage shorn,
The ice on embattlements combs its wake
Hurtles ballasts like quakes under plow stead's
Disputes mud slide chains with daylight frayed stakes
Demeans the lives of anxious quelled fear imbeds,
I think it queer speed ought enforce a code
Repel squid raised turbulent crouched retread
Sequester drapes to hide the enemy's road
Give weighty ire the most cannon distress,
Berate sinister dawn to ranked crustacean
Send light to depths to close eyes which awaken.

Intern 1 :

This day we have been sturdy at the helm
At many islands we found our fame
The torch was lit to host cancers in the realm
Always surgery taxes energy the same,
The briefest storm poured was act a hurricane
Letters carried by pouch were slated indict
Our stay in wet squalor pained the stay
Wounds when knifed put away cold-hearted smite,
Granted children came from the same origin
Whose kin had with infestation joined

Complications wept trials unholy sin
Baskets inbred clung to purple loins,
The rooster flaunts with lust his seedy plum
With tincture reduced by lance and rum.

Intern 2 :

(Stethoscope in hand, enters.)

Terrible howls bespoke with loud mutiny
Sins were betrayed vices clandestine
Shipmates were sent to perform scrutiny
Treat severity by salve of medicine,
Healer's magic unnerved tradition's catch
Branches sawed splints to those who were gloomy
Injections, tourniquets and straps were fetched
Narcotic sensate did whisper entranced roomy,
The nearest isles lay flat by shore geography
Mash units boat procured for massive purge
No epidemic worse to dress choreography
Or make suitable tight skeletons courage,
The grounds were prepared for prophecy
Near-well permitted leave on ship odyssey.

Physician :

Despite fog rolling through mountains made hazy
Tree-tops gave shining sun the tinge of amber
Until all hailed agreed relieved from mazy
Shaded pools were anointed with astound camber,
Eve drafts discouraged clanging bicker
Melancholia imbued with perplex
Dilemma morass by sonorous snicker

Exposure defiled by morbid complex,
We invite exam of ludicrous complaints
Jarring perimeters of capricious doubt
Cogent chastised momentarily restrained
A scholar's custom to train a scout,
A sense of giving away youthful bliss
How to match ends meet a wayward kiss.
We tell ourselves as we mature be personal
Let life not encroach on human domain
Keep at least one intimate friend perpetual
Draw discussion near, bare one's heart abstain,
All circumstance doth contemplate errand
Persuasion adored converts attentive behavior
A life-long trust does take pious retent
Serpent's collar hath lease passion savior,
What caricature must restraint connote
When rainbows at revolt's end are obstructed
Who grafts harvest soddy solemn bestowal
Rumbles rainy barriers roaring object,
Place hands of fate for sentences allotted
Rough coral in sea rebounds in bloody grottos.
Must be the daydreamer strikes to the dimpler
The flapper well is neither redeemed procurer
Fading temper looks fine in receding skimmer
The way fading quibble adjourns to a demurer,
The gust-driven wind may play havoc pelt
Censure inheriting rapine echo
Pluvial rain in sheets revoking spelt
Cast a queer shadow to wed let go,
Inspired downfall tumult tumble to earth
Unreadable carnivores fly about
Inferred deduction recipient berth
Reverberate plural thunder fall out,

Neither the claret nor relapse assign
Complexion a decent compliment sign.

Intern 3 :

(To the Physician.)

Fairly keen to navigate barometer
Perdition perigee, a jilted blast
Spectator flight measured by anemometer
Icy ostracize roar sinewy crash,
Too much aim in ambition that goes wrong
Harsh abandoned new age seeks prime argosy
Pitiable shield for sacred throng
Lament wandering state of havoc cargo,
Lunatic wind erratic needlecraft
Hell bent torment twisted wreck impaired hoax
Suppressed vanities propelling starry raft
Disavow lease, conjure muffled screams coccyx,
Infinite burst induct cradle snowdrift
All life suspended defunct hover air-drift.

Physician :

I can neither say of science gearshift
That society has well served guilt
Except rogue choice entered into by strict
Adherence to prime repented kilt,
These terrors are come upon by occult
Curled frosted sea waves too cold a climate
Impost essentials consecrated for consult
Vaccines and vexed opines knocked chaplet,
Lurid audacious discharged revolver

Neutral unreliable attribute
Defined on X-ray celluloid quicksilver
Like slap shot opium cathode pursuit,
War words with the power to hurt fester
Become intrusive daggers lex non scrpta.
Of matter of conscientious due course
Evolving winds dispute ephemeral moods
Ecstasy depends upon rhapsodic recourse
Billiards berserk once scattered betroth solitude,
This then is the monkey to resolve atoms
Where it coalesces to center form
Tiny legitimacies exerting talons
Nepotisms of quietism anchorite reforms,
Our lives as doctors are to redeem life
We must seek all ramifications first
Liberate cohort from send-off sleep rite
Briefly brave calculate choleric mirth,
It can be added in fewest levies
Yellow gorse strands the binocular bevies.

NURSE :

(Enters.)

Look! I am amazed to find you here
The tow does not impede the ship's careen
But for frozen icebergs in channel fierce
File speed spewing rampant marine,
I quit the task to sew and patch up wounds
Done in time for narcoleptic sleep induce
The crew's reliance kept patients marooned
Until chemist worked prescripts renewed,
I find myself revealed in kindest stoic

Grateful for non-failure organic realize
Low-sodium diet in fish required iodine
Sub-atomic anemia analyzed,
When it would have made sense to minimize
The subject's health caused us to euphemize.

Physician :

I do perceive after twenty years mired
Our ship station received a dozen orders
Cramped quarters and seedy diet strained hires
Good men were drained congealing vertebra,
It occurs time to time our trained habit
Which knows instinct has forgot logic fare
Better men than ours complain of intermit
Carry on gut-bucket style cheeky air,
Fleeting plague, fighting epidemic
Fibrillating fatigue dealt slack of breath
Regiment fever produced mirage pandemic
Bawdy verbose recounted taunt, flaunt and death,
With apparition and depression averted
Intuition and cognition converted.

Intern 1 :

(Uncoils ropes and drops them off side of railing.)

Soon we arrive home to hospice hodden
Gastric edema, melanosis sallow
Orchid organ outgrowth, omens worsen,
Congestion, infarction, mandrel mangled,
Despite the barbarous coast gold lethargy
Visible deformed gangly fractured life

Oncology eclipsed senility
Lymph biopsy mortality midwife,
What must we think about qualified quell
Predictable entropic agility
Benign eyestrain non-sarcoma tell
Rapturous recurrence conviviality,
Diseases that trials of medicine have outrun
Sanctioned healthy tempers by God's triumph.

Nurse :

The ship at sea does appear more closely
While we await to leave for home astern
Systolic system deems the watchful dose
Confides symbolical stillness is learned,
For alcohol alchemy we tried aldosterone
For lashing onset we gave barbiturate
Episodic etymology hormone
Esoteric ego took equilibrate,
The town clinic that shall employ me
Treats bipolar dysfunction at the easel
Eccentric ecclesia with culinary tea
Mild cupidity by restraints feasible,
My sole intent when I first came on land
Assist missions tending infirmed ordinand.
Consternation becomes tedium awake
Where sailors plowshare ends savage dream
That flies the fates of heaven's lonely gate
Arrive hedonist archetype atrium,
Recluse or rescue must by Nature be
Stealth-like attentive to tract movement few
Discerned artifice endeavored internee
While painkiller brokers finder's truce due,

Diagnostician's predisposition aids
Fearful extradition homing
As lance and pierce pellet subdues and fades
Extinguish shock defiant roaming,
Placid bound are instructed for moderate calm
Quiet normalcy returns fate to residual alm.

ACT 5

Scene 1

WIFE :

Simple pleasures restored to Grace's candor
Have wept without end until sustain
Charmed gains knew little of dismal inquisitor
Flights deterred comes round their rightful pertain,
Justice requite borrows its name in bliss
Frankincense steeped in joy denies devise
All cares define marriage with guileless kiss
To bed passion imbues released arise,
I waited over twenty years for you
In vain I struck to join penury forgiven
Despite my age and leisure renewed
With care I sought only what you divined,
To see that you are here at last is reward
I find relief you have my hand life oared.

PHYSICIAN :

I am esteemed in your presence final
A great dismay lifted in all rejoice
That every act was blessed in medicinal
Every prayer subscribed to pledged voice,
I could not wander in fashion approved
Nor studied farthest storm port awakening here
The life and times of one erudite feud
Trenched on hills in guard's leased breath near,
The poor fact rests on merry storms oblige

Despite reasons sent us to oblivion
Merest descript a quest for scarce mirage
Houses removed for plague grand illusion,
Marvels of cleanliness portent refute
Wonders of diet extolled observed dispute.
Were I renounce my pride there would be ear
Enough to find a source of Socrates
Unraveled heard of provinces to steer
The best knowledge accrued by random fees,
Those fines secured in base plucked repartee
Adjoined accounts distilled liquors complete
Abscess did frighten us for wounds to see
I dreamed of you and gave senses reprieve,
It was the dream of life endured afar
That gave me strength to fetch dispense revoked
Not all whose limbs busted may come by war
Not all disgraced review the quest corrupt,
Kindest able kinfolk ought learn remorse
Prayer itself may well find keep in course.
I know after twenty-one year made gone
Like reined horses on snow find food or brine
I grew despaired of returning home long
Took for granted Integrity's soul find,
Faith must in song direct one's solitude
Must seek forgiveness when Fear strides predawn
From east with patterned hoofs charging a feud
Thunderous rumbles strong over the throng,
It is moments like this the earth trembles
The breath takes hold in ice and spends all heat
Keen observance aware retrieves assembles
Cracked bone dormant lies wait for strength to meet,
I should have held these hands for lamps I lit
I had their trust restored in ligaments fit.

You must show me leniency for love
I am naught yet stranger of lives released
If I have not been husband known as glove
I am still home as trust of life aggrieved,
Constance, please know my heart again as found
Try me, my love, endeared medicine grant
The years are young and months endured are bound
Even sky comes with clouds once voices chant,
Tell me our home has swept the cold away
Fate creeds our lost union to winged chariot
Virtues need not agree with starved misplace
Nor sweetest terms debate for long err allot,
My heart has known no risk to worth surmount
Unfix is play until one hears recount.
My sleep doth bid its finest hour employ
I go to chamber stored for leave of grace
Do not attempt to find fracture annoy
Nor take your stay without the hand of day,
For love imbues what it may not dismiss
Cherish awakes the haste it must not crave
Disdain afresh was lost before remiss
And candor spite an eve of care's persuade,
If buds bloomed late in garden's sole remorse
Shed pink and white refrains in winds breezes
As yet a single care I could not store
If wed to you I showed no staying leases,
No maid may take your place in kind to seem
The whole of worlds a thousand words redeem.

(He leaves to bed.)

Wife:

How should I admonish myself implore
That I waited too long and next too brief
Ought I confess I stole a kiss or more
And found solace entwined deployed the keep,
Should I pretend he was the first passion
That not twenty goes by without edict
Surrender does relive the cries rejection
Of time grown cold brings loss heroic,
He gives no clue of what he thinks betrays
Had I his joint wisdom frail scar could rouse
I prefer slow decline of balm belays
Instead of morte that loosens bed drowse,
For good or grief I've hoped to wind a mile
Send home distilled margins of sorrow's guile.
Who waits until the sun has set on grace
Into what state ought my prostrate decline
Wretched boredom the expedition face
First forty I never agreed to sign,
But once of states were wont to complicate
Mare of sixty years in combat I wed
To tempt bellows and church with explicate
Weighty welcome disposed my daily bread,
My son most like his father's mind reflect
Not cares nor leisures does he trim to see
Content to find in company respect
Whereas his son questions any fleur-de-lis,
My creation rises at dawn to draw
Together two as one graph blood rapport.
Only my son's son, full thirty, annoys
Hearsay is wed by lame faults found to grief
Hardly wonder philosopher decoys

Small particles partake average spleen,
His course may not deter the whims of age
To come of sleight disparage stings for fare
Privy in turn gives more a stymied phase
Where sudden grief gives naught a sight of care,
Must age become a state of blessed remake
Must I of guilt demand a case reviled
When shall necessity declare its mate
When may the man come forth who gave the child,
If Charity displayed rightful heir son
Ought life rejoined be kept or be redone.
Singularity a stoic branch of life
Creates the worth of days apart by sums
Who shall announce the start of major rife
Who knows as well the thunderous played drums,
Vaccines may quell a titanic title
Thieving thieves dress the roles spoilage
Consensual bargains repair requital
Matrimony duplicitous hostage,
Passage grants passenger a ticket shorn
Of kind mapping sea fraught predicate earned
Reducible reality forlorn
Heaven to life appreciative preen exturned,
Not careful or cautious has acts unseen
Legal and liable restrict not foreseen.

Son :

(Enters.)

We sat to lunch and ate discourse through charts
It seemed apparent the injured men denied
The thrift of allegiances profound risked starts

Last gasp by foolish clutch were judged belied,
Like those worst dreams versions of Achilles heel
Creeping spiny acanthus herb stagnate
Glimmers emitting light sparks gathered black steel
Abdications purpose accumulate,
Corrosive trickery most habitual
Downcast obsessions ripe deceived desserts
Effigies strung like wicked vines residual
Dank vain declivities gave chase to myrrh's,
Lack of moral virtue an absent craft
Vigorous inhibitions gushed with graft.
Why waste the mortal body fair of rank
Covet harm's spree to enshrine weak express
Dozen cases asserted divested gangplank
Favor dispelled conveyed unrestrained aggress,
Entire conspire of tense cataclysm
Joined flaunt frolic beside wet blades baited
Hindered finite acts to heal incision
Gave suspicions composed ardent created,
The fact that medicine should be agreed
Not berated morsels convened for luck
Record-keeping left bay for vestments read
Miserable campaign distorted brief muck,
Only reliable creatures sparkled
Admirable inquests described usable.

Constance :

(His mother; Wife.)

You are hard pressed to view the mort while clear
Abhor absence of health before succumbs
Deny rushing whistle as breath loses dear

Abandon dark missions to event thumb,
Supine stupor symbiotic weak swoon
Clandestine harpsichord a ballad awake
That hears the suffering sweet sick tune
And bribes heaven or hell with swift dull stake,
To gaze upon forelocks briefly entire
Give spoon a bitter vile to drench spirit
Indolence cost its own inference sire
Take pulse every dark hour for naught queered,
Life leaves marrow shallow promise
Discards comfort to ill's squalid darkness.

Son :

(Takes her hand, kneels.)

I beseech you, tell me what dad requires
You know his moods, his dreams, knowledge, finds
I can no more disturb his sleep or spire
I feel I must summon his eye and mind,
Consecrate blight to an acrid exile
A vigilant watch of tremulous life
Purify rampant venereal lifestyle
Preserve fertile defeat against gripe,
Augment by skill gauze ligature permit
Control leukocytes, tolerate fatigue
Test scarlet fever with Dick, Schick for dip
Wasserman syph, basal metab agree,
Did he suggest reclassify defect
Did he theorize the mind deficit?
Does he prefer stricken or stoppage yield
Terms of scourge dew upon stallion splash hills
May I suggest extrude for atrophy

When skies teemed with rain contradict wills,
Saccharin crop lies fluted with rabid mash
Wind through vine fields flutter vibrant alive
Conquerable stress makes vibrating lash
Defibrillate degeneracy thrive,
Help me, Mother, in smit moonlit couplet
Narcotic trauma aided by dose sucrose
Addict torment inflicts his own conflict
Screenings absolve the abscess indispose,
Am I mistaken to want his approval
Ailment altered secures kind removal.

CONSTANCE :

Please stand, my son, there is no necessity
Expedition travel assures protect
Succeed you must to unclasp corsetry
Redesign incuse a mandatory object,
Could I given you a sibling welcome
To acclimate nomenclature reason
I would never refuse series postmortem
Nor assassinate cooperation season,
Far be it for me to deny you love
Absent version its unrestrained purpose
Abdicate innovate, deviate truelove
Steer stellar fortification syllabus,
My advice is borrow your whims for fate
Defer judgment until compounds illuminate.
The ways of flesh propagate far to know
Distinct release infuse the mind blessings
That life holds dear the best promises bestow
Weather fortune purple amaranth owing,
Catling or sling must take obliging loathing

Describe in charts picturesque frost of grip
Foster unfriendly fence by comfort bathing
Dispel weakness of heart excepting equip,
Your father corks scaffold endears binding
He blends contrite divest in armored sheaths
Confines those ill to helpless finite nursing
Stabbings, rasping, gas veined, cocoons all wreaths,
Pertain to his unique cohesive courses
Become like him in practiced resources.

Son:

I may tell you we spoke of moron greed
The sort festers in fruit of all gestation
Unsuspecting youth suffers viscous speed
As veteran rancor and hated vexation
Create a fog of invisible movement
Ruffle a rising virulent nest swarm
Massacre hills breathe insects imminent
Unyielding multitudinous cruciform,
Like diseased pickled roe incurrent slain
Reprehensible vermin mangled wings
Blackened hillsides choking in carnage plain
Translucent wasps muffled in muddy stings,
Transpired spinning murmurs like spitting hail
Unsympathetic dung spattered in Braille.
He was worst affected by this heinous ravage
Day eclipsed by horrid assailing sounds
A mummery myriad riddles savage
In which men's voices were fragmented drowns,
They charged every which way mullets drawn
Their boots sinking through rotten vines long vexed
Nested blood having replaced flowing thorn

Sickeningly pungent the sour scent vested,
If this were symbolic rather than scene
I might think twice of heretic spoils
I am convinced the celestial nadirs bring
Wood legs, fract spines, heat strokes, sweat, mindless toils,
An emerging pestilence grown of sweet leisure
Sufficient hail flying at wind liberator.

Constance :

Were such mania true it comes unbearable
To not recognize in advance the shores
Rancid humor lies below ease as cable
Twisted vine which assembles flimsy bored cores,
Destructive rails imprint a man's footfall
His sense provides no overture of land
Repeated yields construe mental volleyball
Chagrin promised duty even on sand,
Vigor most promised stealth that curtails doves
It tricks the mind aspects of immortal
Incestuous groves haunted in decked whisked roves
Not all governed by tolerant portal,
Steady as she bellows the port is near
Although gardens untamed fetch honey fear.

Son's son :

(Enters.)

I could not hear the total measure lost
At guess chartreuse willow alters window
A day of hail produces months neglect frost

Snow piles abound too deep to find the crow,
Merry slaughter forbids its trench to grow
Avenues creaked run foul afield glimpse
The heart that finds its path glutted by tow
Branched marrow a view finder's quits,
Sorrow is the harmed rant for bloomed carcass
Despite gullible ill findings adjourned
Winter furrows like spring tide marked harness
Soapy dew drops incline marsh woods sod fern,
Glassy glaucoma doth shine mirrors deceit
Thwarted glaciers underfoot tremble delete.

Son :

(His father, laughs.)

Humor in essence weds the pain to gaff
Retrieves sanity to its rightful foot
The bramble land skewers distilled draft
Laudable lariat supplies opium root,
It shows when we converse the healing words
Friendship supports our ailing reminisce
Even with your mother removed our mirth
Forgives questions about neglect's abyss,
I see you wrote your grand a fine address
Pretty pictures of us at Plymouth beach
It put him right at home God bless your press
Reduced the years and placed them in his reach,
This week we three will board the ferry to Cairns
Weigh salt and train to Melbourne's renown quern.

ACT 5

Scene 2

(Constance and Friend in the park.)

CONSTANCE :

This is farewell, my friend, my husband is home
Deceit I shall not woo despite contents
I am sworn that he never learns tome
Although I know kindness repays relents,
I have employed his young mistress for play
My grandson's laugh betrays slovenly time
He casts queer lights about to mistake fey
He broods of threats for power's secret rhyme,
I know my limits fair reply resign
I ought discern that quests for truth gamble
A heady torque that stays rebuke's design
You may advise but love denies ramble,
Your ring I give to you of intended aim
May I not place that tryst to slay disdain.

FRIEND :

Beware rebukes that sting are merely claims
Enhance your faith in splendorous rejoice
Negate the whims desired plague remains
Enter medicine, it's the better voice,
Heed grace, live pure, restore guileless encounter
No one has seen the low remiss enjoined
Could be that all he means is mixed flounder

A felled misstep that breaches mistrust coined,
It should not be a sharp dagger misused
Nor blade rusted breath beneath one's skirt
Simple betrayals are trials abused
Sonorous thoughts decry intention's girt,
I shall always be found waiting reply
I live for you surrendered delight.

Constance :

I do not imagine this tryst for you
Would not subscribe you to this wretched act
Were my husband not barren I would have few
No pride have I secrets to implore the fact,
Yet keen I am possessed of knowledge disgraced
Besides you two I keep no pleasure stoked
To Purity I maintain more love faced
No heartaches climbed do I wish to cloak,
Fear makes no entrance where I reside safe
My son's son may outgrow his nimble rebel
Yet how many breaths shall I hold for chaste
When love's honest doorstep dreams cannot quell,
Entrust to you accomplice will for life
My only god spell primed bribery's knife.

Friend :

(Aside.)

Such foresight, brilliant intelligence, are we
Here come to despair?

(To her.)

I pray for you, Constance, that you lack sight
This folly has no febrile constancy
It mends no grace to God's hand in right
Stifles the very air with immunity,
Shall I say naught to Eduard who deserves
The err of one baleful night to slay
Passions of task too brief to know of purge
Less servile choice to comfort execute stay?

CONSTANCE :

I hate myself worse than I can lie
You know not love to say I might approve
Fatal charms castigate a roving eye
Boredom has recompense in horror's brood,
I saw no choice conceived of blood relation
Win him over without infestation
May Fate not crow at thirsty elation
Nor meddle irk the foregone conclusion,
His father, my son, is all I keep
Worship the day of birth his fallacy
If his father knew he was barren he reaped
And I my place begot a family,
I am not a greedy minded zealot elf
Although that harlot wed my son mislaid
Her ballad her son repeats since he was twelve
Interprets at every turn a nasty craze,
The screws are tight with artifice
My father-in-law entrusted his will an heir
Which leaves idle pleasures requisite risk
I won't bother with vain apology tear,
Could I have made a life of pleased refine
Congestion strait jacket would yield design.

FRIEND :

I implore you to act with judicious wit
It's shown folly is her weapon unkind
Delivers a blow resounds its blade herewith
Gives none the sight of petty smite made blind,
We could of course repair to meet sometimes
To spoil hourly savors enlisting day
Broker advantage less the night reclines
Draft torn wayward advance until we may,
Let us resolve no injury apart
Nor felled avarice injunct for heaven's prayer
It is schooled years that find graces of art
And fools hurt whims that take passion's aim dare,
Do not dispose of love and plead remorse
Or darken civility with undue course.

CONSTANCE :

I must assert my oaths before sunset
Disguise merit to rake the wheel astern
Twenty aged years remain subscribe neglect
When sons ought come with sons proper return,
I will not squelch our family tide
Break bread by slaying descendent history
The moon doth rise at equator's first bide
Its light silvery blue casts rays blustery,
I should remove a gleam which tricks the cards
And prune the rose thorns of bloodied winced prick
Perjure the easy man his vent of shards
Earthen his wares by throwing him his stick,
Philosopher-doctrined shall he earn pay
Knowledge kept wound refit his labours haste.

Friend :

We each have fantasies of spite in mind
Which takes a toll on exhaustion stymied
That weigh fortune destined with comfort chimed
Sit weary time to breathe verses keyed,
Over fifty seasons we have conversed
Looked upon the fates with aged relief
Struck change for perfection wed redeemed curse
Solaced lover's charmed knots in failed belief,
Returned before to now again release
We tell ourselves it's all for good portend
The son half mine knows naught of time's poor grief
Sorrow may chide regret yet sends surrend,
Nothing rejoiced spent lasts eternity
That we enlist their lives for true earnesty.

(Lights fade for a moment; as dim lights come on, Friend is gone and Illusion is with her.)

Illusion :

At last we stand together foe and heart
I have waited almost a life to speak
Shall hope be made a port for hatred's part
Faulty perception fused deceit fair cheek?
We are neither kind meant as beast or tree
We walk, possess, have choice, free will and sail
We come to life and by misfortune weak
Do heed the call of peril break through storm gale,
When right and wrong suffer loss of value
Call on redemption save our mortal souls
Wail! Wail! Barely in form a mirage blue

I rise spirit from flesh as ill takes tolls,
I am neither Virtue or Quality
Life must have conscience and purity.
Who has not committed crime starts with Virtue
My sisters are Charity and Mercy
Ideals make society's base, Virgil's due
States four grieved sins that kill, hate and envy
Worse than willful penury and adultery
Disloyal to conscience, chosen destiny
Not relief destiny, your despair pair-y
You are remote headed for life's brevity,
Your crime to snare the husband's heart ought leave
For basic life as Socrates describes
A place to live, some food, healthy wreath
Attire and shoes and job prison imbibes,
Despite Pilapaedis food for lotion to cure
As physician you must contend with lure.

Constance :

How else do I save my son from harm
My husband cannot live on army pay
His blessed virtue to be primary farm
His life is chosen for wounded stay,
How do I get my grand to retract his aim
Plot point recourse to the farthest star
His thoughts like his mother before him feign
Follow each whim or chart an oar too far,
Shall he impede husband's loving design
Act of malice injure grievous nurture
Will he succeed in declarations resign
A greed that seeks a wound to boast demure,
I shan't repeal intent or permit boasts to bloom

This house belongs to me in earnest plume.

ILLUSION :

You are not weak without moral revision
You may arrive in mind to slew your slate
You ought retreat the starting incision
Harness your sights to fields of rain abate,
View wrath as killing pestilence denied
Water when drunk may quench desire at first
Prescribe a dose legal to chase one's pride
Only by fault might we gamble the purse,
Intangible dagger thrust deep to his breast
Reviled language to dress the fool's costume
Imparts the fist that beats the door aggress
Sorely wanders the storm's thunderous tomb,
I came because I heard your friend lament
The trust of love defies courage descent.

ACT 5

Scene 3

(Husband is reading a book in the sitting room, Constance enters.)

CONSTANCE :

You must think me an utter coward tamed
To have thrust me husband's mistress so crude
Tortured mistrust have you petty to blame
To think I could befell the worlds remove,
This house longer remains to spill most fates
Destiny relief conjures a prim disguise
Deplores even catching fever distrait
Matters sincere reduced for envy's lies,
Renee may be a pretty thief of time
May spend a suture's worth in shamed retort
For which is love and which is queer refine
Wherein convenes conscience practiced distort,
At least I rest on laurel vines convey
I make my bed on chaste ideals of day.

HUSBAND :

No pretty face has she to compare to you
Nor fairer words extol medicine be sung
Or found redundancy pertain your rue
Or woo fancy ambition a balm undone,
Who asks of you the ways of love to scorn
When you feed on jealous insufficiency

We know you made the lotions where you were born
The time and date when you achieved decree,
You do not add productive reason heard
Nor dispatch regard of your sought hurry
Should you attempt to mark your state by word
Who could decrease your tempest veal worry,
It gnaws at me to hear distress forlorn
As though you earn estate by light's foghorn.

Constance :

I quest an heir to free your average fate
Stood proud to ken a magnitude
Intern Robert swore no return contemplate
Your will set free your valor rescind feud,
If I be faithless blamed you accrued foresight
Love torn apart holds no fare completed to
That I share gains you have no face at night
Divest rightful possession gleaned allude,
Removed by rank a wife is sure a slave
Life sleeps to breathe the love that Man adores
I walked to altars for my only grave
I know not how your words can come restores,
Promises are few to compete with tears wept
Joint vows may not live up to charmed descript.

Husband :

It was a mere remark that chanced a lamb
I gave you day and fine repay spoils
In all my hours I am yet here a man
Whose father spared me his finest toils,
In his discharge I stayed my sharpest grief

Forgave his errs and described myself port
I knew while he deceased depart I keep
My true resolve became my living court,
Why shan't you live with heaven's folly
Ought I look to your awes with joined relief
Console my days without esteem idly
Brandish design as though it were a chief,
Who loves yet once to know complaints regain
Returns relieved that kin foster abstain?

Constance :

Then shall I speak plainly the purchase rout
How can I go on if you leave again
What shall I think – even ten years raise doubt
I may endure nightmares of truth to learn,
Approve you gone begrudge your whim to flee
Consecrate all my faith in your absence
Charmed life elsewhere ingests a hard envy
How could you do this lie to me incense?

Husband :

Why start to falsify choices you have made
I can no more answer untimely blows
Than adhere to generous fault misplaced
My love waits here with kindest woes.

Constance :

I will feel duped, word gets around
How many times will I not know the key
Must I resent your journeys abound

Shall I inquire has she better than me,
Loathe the surgery she shall duty perform
Embark on chores repent forfeit power
Seek naught my sworn chalice surfeit inform
Give thanks for you to leave early tower,
Become a nag who winces at every thought
Worry you may think cause to leave perchance
Disclaim Reason as thought it were a draught
Take bed to find in sleep I keep a chance,
A rift shall sorely prove withdraw our bond
To have to part with the mate I respond.

Husband :

(Gets on bended knee.)

Connie, you cannot wish to invite force
You have no pleas permit digression
No deck hand lives for least intercourse
Nor aim to charge unfit obsession,
It is impaired to seek love lost sentries
Quite the reverse, overlook our small tomb
Enjoy our life together without entreaties
It is my right that you remain my wound,
I heal your recants in return for acceptance
My sole trespass my sin to deny death
Pastures of dying men in prayer's trance
Nothing more can I say to implore breath,
You must eternal know you are my deed
My light in oceans of forests decreed.

Constance *(to Illusion)* :

You may consider my pleas impotent cries
A thousand wise pardons do not decrease
It is not just matters of indulgent dies
That I should find my nights offered release,
You may inquire whom I sent her to keep
Aware will slack a blade to the breast fed
Butcher the keen mistake for no lasting reap
Refrain from tasks as time might amend bread,
Demand I must before I wake for light
Decry my fate to be filled worse with hate
Only protect my life against mourned blight
Destroy the man who wrote obliged of late,
Govern disgrace by any hand or clamp
Disease him to the Winds of carrion stamp.

Illusion :

Wail! There is no turning back agreed
Bequest yourself a new relation impound
You give yourself no safe port anchor seek
The worst has yet to sift the dour found,
Wail! Vile treachery is afoot
Aggrieved remarks shall give offense dispute
Misfortune takes the poisoned arrow root
Makes all retire language object refute,
Tell him what you have done to enlist minds
Do instruct him your cast of clay is harsh
Release yourself of spent passive binds
Event query cannot restore seed to marsh,
Go now! Destiny forbids one's able starve
Charity depleted grants further larvae.

ACT 5

Scene 4

(Son John and his father William who is Husband in garden.)

JOHN :

Laurence has found a bride to marry him
Her name is Renee and she is nurse to Army
He states she is unlike any female limb
Quite capable, pretty, endowed in purity,
I said I would ask you for your blessing
He thinks a faire addition to the family
She lacks fertility although may bring
Any fare you could design anomaly,
I have agreed invite to Melbourne town
Tour city life and shore by night and day
Provide cottage and keep clubs gun and gown
Train ride to Cairns and board a boat in quay,
Such enjoyment attribute to crescent
Treasured advance on Whidbey Islands rent.

WILLIAM :

(To himself.)

At last I view the open graves are paved
I fear Constance distress may be worsened
Neglect to Laurence if I seem depraved
A kiss of war doth wend its way descend.

(To his Son.)

At last the card is thrown by fate bestow
I could not allow rejection to deny
Of course we will celebrate years unfold
Arrange anchor and yard to house his bride,
Tell him that every summer we sail
Hobart by yacht with masts flying in wind
Speed race to point along stone cliffs of Braille
Steer fate to win the title furl upwind,
Spent time carries the jib like skis on ice
Breakneck instinct handles the ropes in seconds
Winded regret defies brave course its tithe
Refuse would be unkindly cleaving wrongs,
Bring forth the rice and we will break the glass
To chart a ship philosopher his brass.

JOHN :

I am relieved your blessing is divined
We shall set course for evening's shallow tide
To walk the beach with flowing ribbons twined
Follow the sea until the moon full shines,
I shall invite Hazel just this once joy
Flowers into the waves starling a strewn
Footprints on black sloped sand enjoy
A din of bats as tide restores pools stream,
Melbourne seaweed red horns in mud equipped
Dispute the ocean roar visitant lathe
Bulbous cacti distract tintypes grip
Dark sky, sea rinsed brown flats tinted bathe,
We each require penitential sorrel
Vestal recreation to uncoil slip's chapel.

William :

I wonder how we may revisit eudemonics
Happiness stemmed after virulent war
Considers pharmaceuticals with geoponics
Potato, baize, stalk and root consist of oar,
Tryptophan or valerian root tea
Next Zen combines with therapeutic mend
Peaceful being to cope effectively
Traduce the brain's mortality transcend,
We ought not leave unsaid transparency
Tragedian complexes tread on traits
Enmeshed paucity redacts congruity
Violent emotion the autopsy of distrait,
Man's fidelity not less impiety
Sobriety quenches anxiety.
Can we be said human we are humble
Without debility we are spousal?

John :

Contrivance disposes men to weak aim
Lacerates cofferdams in diabolic sin
We must arrive before damage takes claim
Digitalis, mercury, hemlock all poison,
What are humans about besides latent
Vulgarism, recidivism, nepotism
Why are we not more trying resistant
Fatalist analysts suffering occultism,
Who can determine if the hand may strike
Aerialists fly before the net is hung
Do invectives cause pain before a knife
Fever emit after the bell is rung?

What must I read to comprehend gain
Restraint which binds or those reins that attain?

ACT 5

Scene 5

(Laurence and his father John.)

LAURENCE :

Renee departed the marriage late in the month
She said the fun aboard the yacht oppressed
She thought that aim for misery did front
Although the maiden voyage did give rest,
I pled she make the cottage yard her garden
I said I am a patient man by far
It was not her intent to flirt warden
Or sign my wit for Whidbey's farthest shore,
I have remorse that I cannot marry
My star leaves home to travel alone
What part of my mother do I tarry
Which part of you bears witness tasks keystone?
I loved this girl with all my heart declared
When we turned wheel into the wind, what fared?

JOHN :

No better I explain a female's mind
It frocks pending elusive hopes apace
With time flourishes true a great design
Your mother was cautious with no efface,
Reverse duress, my son, worries depress
Perchance displaced bootlace gave her false verse
One day you will find beckoned love endless

If she is not the one others traverse,
Thirty you are yet a young man afoot
Life starts when grant tenure installs a lease
Feckless attract grows impatient rebut
Chariot's report may wish teacher to please,
You are alarmed by hurt that she overlooked
There is no one to blame, she was not hooked.

Laurence :

What does father think, a wink of sleep has he
I dare say naught if he caught a hasty turn
With all there is to do prepare splint fees
He must have lost a night to learn
I did enjoy the bit of wit esteemed
I heard the news recap the world plight
Rolex yacht cup, prime minister and team
Winged insects scourge was rampaged with blight,
Will grand transcribe expedition day charts
Shall he require counts high fever, weak strain
Number metabolic disorder, malaria hearts
Count pyaemia, leucopenia scrape
I could assist records as to causes
Decreased penury suppress luckless.

John :

Of course Father thinks you shall most restore
The future year looks bright for hospice seer
The hand to prescribe health against abhor
May be blessings researched to end great fear,
I want to be certain your studies on Mind
Occur as well you live assured at Mel

Summers may bring drops of rain to find
Sorrows tender abide proper pain quelled,
Graduation before college instruct
Shall give the best relief a life enjoy
Best live at school than find obstruct
Perils of Socrates must grant employ,
If all is known we advance by design
For that which we are taught a Self define.

Constance :

(Enters.)

There you are, John, Father wants you at once
I fear you have neglected his serum ward
He thinks the scourge fevers are plied with dunce
He asks that you prepare his tea to bard,
I know you wish Aspects to stand with grace
To pine mortal enmeshed disease to leave
The late hour becomes a fine limb state
Governed distraught bequests a studied wreathe,
Opal discerns jaundiced facial remorse
Pallor aggrieved belies the look of blue
The ears are tried by rings to dismal force
The heart borrows heavy quiet mouth rue,
A son's wonder escapes a brief release
That stays a life for elegant surcease.

John :

(Takes his mother's hand.)

Your hand is cold, I fear the wind does bleat

The sad regret of Patience rests upon your brow
The leaves are strewn by eve's hurried pale feet
A storm defies the sharpest skies endow,
Do keep few words for Laurence whose fancy
Detached her rope from height of mast unfurled
He struck a pinnacle with hopes dancing
He gave his soul to her lyrical world,
She left without so much a word forward
After promised address of future dreams
If you may speak to his preened attuned sard
Relieve distress of unkindly bound seams,
Answer his call for wretched part desire
Allow compassionate winds chase retire.

(He exits.)

Constance :

Laurence, you went on a black fool's errand
The footing fleet of my husband's privy
Medicine doth pretend to lure fair send
He revealed love more absolute priory,
Renee disclosed a bard resound affair
Hiked skirt thus high for his immoral touch
An intern informed me by letter care
Described liaison o'er two years approached clutch,
I was given descript of their remorse
Hundred insects flying above their breasts
The taint offends a foul odor discourse
Blackens the earth with horrible small pests,
To imagine duty like fond repair
Harbored instinct pastures lifeless ensnare.

Laurence :

You must be wicked to send me cruel grief
Only hatred in your heart destroys its prey
Had I any treacherous thought how brief
You send dispatch murdered rage to pay,
Who would you be to have the stage of spite
Relate or die or quench your lover's kiss
You grieve before you live to conquer life
Forgive your barren soil a feigned bliss,
Marriage of hours unholy crease record
Find one mate tried corporeal parity
Were I fashioned of mankind's nary discord
I should find you a dark polarity,
Sane deeds keep loyal friends in harmony
Accomplices abound in keen alacrity.

Constance :

Spare me unwise selfish caprice and affair
You who are yet at college ambition
Dwelling at home under our protective fare
Library or research, neither gives rendition,
Sadly, sickly or madly or badly
We placed you in Cairns to study epidemics
You make a spoony lad for philosophy
Too much proven are you a maverick;
While you succeed listening to Puccini
How many years of study is twenty
Worthwhile endeavor is sublimely untimely
Neglect tracheotomy, gastronomy
One day you may succumb to Houdini
Become a veritable destiny of ignominy.

LAURENCE :

Had I but one jawbone for sedition
I ought confess a nature repudiate
Nomenclature a telling repetition
Eradication of allergy a mutate,
The prey in hand doth extinguish bowers
As readily the trilogy tradition
May bring final graduation cowers
Quested accrued allergy ambition,
My love imposed upon to ill design
Proscribes the writ too foul feudal scheme
Criticism borrows debate resign
Before gambol debacles a vital mean,
Cynicism reduces tangible rank to seethe
Where strife asserts clovers bequeath.

CONSTANCE :

Bluster unseen cannot harbor regret
When best is yet a promised net redact
Buckle secured relieves future forget
Thumb plucked plumage grows thin prologue abstract,
I gave your revision phantom pharmacy
Pantomime played like Romeo removed
Virtuous doom argued morphology
Your sane Mother ushered mortgage accrued,
Virgil civil code trivial philander
Pillaging pillory constricts pigment
Ontogeny beneficent pillar
Decides prejudiced pipe aroused stigma,
Adjourn domestic providence maxim
Frugality prolonged customs quorum.

LAURENCE :

Diligent repartee raison d'etre
Manageress of acquisition stress
Father purchased a cottage in Mel fair
Rancid malice revives fury aggress,
Although rampage makes disgrace sharp with shame
Your rebuttal distributes far chaos
No normal sense have you restraint regain
The house keeps ears for all ethos,
Distill essence life never imparts dross
Disturbs relate as well the heart portends
My father in charity grants no loss
Despite haven true allusion depends,
Which hand compass doth find verbose deceits
To err sport upon hung ravens deletes.
That generosity engraves all Time
Virology extends cardiology
Guised eulogy retort makes haste its rhyme
How quick the sick must deign harmony,
Agony brief litany strung portrays
Sirens cavort in specious arrogance
Cacophony completes golden sunrise arrays
Clucky reticence doth sting jurisprudence,
Abroad a host of moors distinguish read
Banal, puerile subjects inform defense
Whereas schooled art insures the mind its keep
For jail insult disowns academy intent,
Sagacity reforms device usage
Unreal measure lacks true divine carriage.

CONSTANCE :

I acknowledge the incongruity
Incidental indebted contest incurred
Dystrophy brings great absence dignity
Forty years at sea bears no cost disturbed,
Who are you to judge my infertility
Why ought you to define my gauge remorse
Should I explain the lack of mortality
If years pronounce their sense remiss discourse,
Hazel like you upset my quiet refrain
Followed every footstep into kindness
Whose money ought be released disdain
With all impedes as if the store were blessed,
You make your bed among your chosen finds
Leave me and mine to view the sun inclined.
Know naught your age for whom the toll deprives
Thirty is too youthful to have austere
Alter rivers to wend their way to lives
Pretend you hear decent hallows nervure,
Counsel knowledge before you set your quest
Love fast as you intend to die in vain
Erect your house on firm soil for rest
Try hard to learn Heaven on earth arraign,
Vacancy of breath shows relation
Varnish may appear rued by grain reduced
Adhered cocoon sheds once fine invention
Narcotic drug cyclone atones seduced,
Red matador arrests the beast for prize
Until transgress repair the lark's disguise.

(William enters)

William :

Here we are revealed in plurality
My two favored redemptions to living
Your father John shall bring you to the sea
I agreed purchase nearest your believing,
Arrive by day to stay the whole of thought
Enjoin morning to Rolex winsome cup
Latent conjure its sweetest briar sailcloth
Describe amidst coral twine nets scup,
Placid reference rejuvenates won
Contemplation of study defines the hour
Colloquy heard ponders Regard anon
Argument in Lord Courts describe the bower,
Obscurity observed belies foundation
From which Death rigors predict lexicon.
One esteemed autumn describe the Aspects
Contradict worse Envy and Greed pertain
Intent to kill, bribery, deed remove, affects
Joint nurse, cunning extrapolate feign,
Informed consent, predate medication
Sworn document, defiled estate function
Reduced morte with spoiled serum solecism
Lithograph parsimony obscured Assumption,
Roman Law is descript for Charity
Relate becomes the physician's rarity.

Laurence :

Most kind a word you give to me in grace
I could not wont better findings conveyed
In sum wanderings late appear of state
Whence none gave Will a veil of Fate,

I shall oft think Eros defines arrow
Bestowed with Grace the sea brings life anew
Green fields rejoice the sun and moon allow
More apt a sailor's risked life completes for few,
Ready to leave I ought shine marksman's prow
Discern the clay of which Mankind is made
Bear charts ignored Psyche to restore endow
Probate distract lessons of contemplate,
I take my leave to walk the path imbued
Trials of drought must surely end construed.

(He exits.)

WILLIAM :

You have taken my heart from me for fun
Showered petals of ire about the sand
Virulent storms aggress with each redone
Until alas I am found out a puny rand,
You keep a man for John to know his prayer
Suffer I do in haste to perceive my state
I have endured the aims of fate for lair
No gains shall seek into the goodly bait,
Should you encroach upon our happy wed
As yet I shan't provide you with a dime
Expect complete fealty in our bed
Without implore decide our love a crime,
If you must see this man I shall abandon
Make you a sty and opine your tryst sun.

CONSTANCE :

You heard my words without reality

Stole hope from trust for randy limb too plain
He is your closest match who knows your pleas
Exhibits all those cares to inhibit sane,
Intend I must to give your loyal kiss
No breath will take our son away to sea
You shall endear yourself as sex to bliss
Promise tender foot renewed entreaty,
Without your love I grow coldly absent
No shadow will I keep between our hours
Nor take a spoon of draught enjoined in rent
Or hide my grief alone discouraged dours,
I claim all you require in footing and breath
You shall deny the past regret to death.

WILLIAM :

(Arm around her shoulders.)

Dearest Constance, neglect your pithy wit
Desire only have I in past for you
A trust of share no paradox befit
Were we to part company precise reduce,
Parallax ought no impairment be seen
Ideal paradigm echoes with jealous truce
Winds blow lashing my roads prolong esteem
At last quiet inveighs mortal refuse,
Walk me along garden delights once more
Forgive the past burdens enchanted hillsides
Endure stellar optimism implore
Fasten rigid splint save fracture besides,
Steer me, coax me, intoxicate infect
Shore me to hours punish fledgling distress.
Logic converts witchcraft ignite negate

Downfall maintains immoral coin obverse
Judgment kindly baffles sleeping opiate
Testy expense owing mythic traverse,
Moonlight hemoglobin pillory expose
Badger wretched husband whose only worth
Falls free appointed post degree bestows
Elixir craft medicate for smart mirth,
Collude with me in whole matrimony
Rigor the love extrapolate vignette
All goods that claim our son likely guaranty
Matchless excel salver justice pundit,
Suspend my life by celestial polestar
Inform again repeat sweaty spark spar.

(Stage lights fade.)

ACT 5

Scene 6

(Garden scene Physician and Son)

Physician :

Life has taken a most sorrowful turn
Your mother stays another winter abroad
Salty Cairn winds provide a spate astern
Despite fractured solace portend distraught
She writes whimsy sends no forked remark
Café museums distill complacent breeze
Evening chill hosts studied canoes in stark
Lit apparitions spar fluid leaves ease
Diaphanous blue waves assure marked Time
Repetitive clinging traces footprints on sand
Day decreases under brush strokes design
Mulled wine discerns the ablest mere strand,
Who may relate isolation's demise?
The heart heavy stains tears in darkest sighs.
Briefest hours confide the swiftest Mind
Briefer Psyche astute forgives replies
Deeply perceived convent spackles the bind
Sudden parity enmeshes denies,
This makes our first major separation
I have been patient as best I may be
For Love's trials are mere connotations
Described to seldom erred relief to keep,
Palpations faint increase the store regret
Acceptance brings about kindly reprieve

Years apart have taught us to know asset
Forgiveness steers by its star as it grieves,
She asked that you come as soon as permits
Before night shadow creases intimate.

Son :

My mother is my soul; for her I rest
Sentiment waits until she restores trust
Her reluctance keeps for my selfless quest
I know as Good enjoins Charity adjust,
Constance shall return to health to assist
We will meander along seacoast and town
Speak humor and satire in terms aorist
Devote mirth to appraise complaint's frown,
I will say I miss her here, I am aimless
I cannot imagine studies to proceed
The time goes slowly in spite of our bless
The farthest shore seems farther yet decreed,
Silly parent whose son maintains keen hours
To where has love gone astray in her glower?

Physician :

I miss her too, long hours keep me awake
Wondering if I ought travel to her
Manacle tradition as library drake
Matriarch peculiar prefer,
Keepsake memory vigorous decline
Bestow genius invective medicine
Reach for love's reunite as holy sign
Without wasted mortal leased sin,
I miss our family late gatherings

All rebukes, laughter and recitals fare
Frippery, despicable eavesdropping
Latitude, heraldry, prudent bare,
Frequent gadabout pet midnight mischief
Old topper, sweet gregarious rampage.

Son :

I thought you and I might boat the rain
Sidney this time of year easy entry
To rent a yacht, mast wind, trim raw brown cane
Sturdy on an island, drink swill, camp brie,
Few days in sun, girth alligator by cut
Take Mom dancing, corsage orchid, big blue sea
Snorkel, snap photo, fry squid, sleep in, strut
Converse, read newspaper, make her a plea
Cottage next door ---

Physician :

We may visit morrow if you wish
Leave our day work to coastal Australia
See our Constance flurry about replenish
Amuse ourselves in her comfort and folly,
Bring cheer, step in fashion, adhere grief
So much the wane eve tide rushes to shore
A kite flying to catch a passing breeze
Ferry across inlet, grassy dunes store,
Merit totem, bestow finer hours
Proffer quick wit and manage traverse path
Sit by the window sill while waves lour

Read Dante in bed amid fluttering sash,
Frozen peach popsicles, day old blue sheets
Broken wall clock skipping more than a beat.
My life weighs no disappointments unclear
No oars removed, the boat moored for weather
We ask ourselves, how far into the steer
As flocks overhead describe the wide feather,
Is there ample succumb to fall to earth
Is joy prescript denied when chants row ships
Does Male find malcontent disagreeable berth
Shall Age wander afar to sting kissed lips,
Palomino like quest bolts swift on course
Ears pinned, it flies afield, avows moonlight
Scrimmages sultry findings perforce
Mischievous penury tosses deadlight,
If foresight stows rational Interrogate
Must ice frostbite cohort Inoculate?

INTERN 1 :

(Enters),

Your vessel, Sirs, has arrived to seaport
Shall you deport before the eve regrets
I have recipient warrant for court
Sequent Trieste ship's rope holdfast arrest,
We deport in Melbourne by early light
Windswept black beach littered by mud marsh stones
Set forth by van to north permafrost blight
Poltergeist morns and spiny finned fish bones,
Life faith assured for post mort lust missive
Positive cortex journey comes to delve
Imprint distinct productive salve passive

Improves adaptive thrive for trove involve,
In two days hence the hedge soap trees shall bloom
Silver red buds break poems canons entomb.

Son :

You made our plans without telling me first
I am so elated I scarcely breathe
I have parted a hundred tears of worst
Pricey chance I mistook piety,
Come, dad, let's grow tipsy on efficiency
Charity its own reduction finds plain
Sanity after sleep relieves lethargy
Decipher languor, rigger the toss mane,
Hinder the calendar until the jib
Crosses deck and sails free on salty air
Fiddler coddler gambler paddler bib
Release a knowing worth in pander's fare,
We stand at trim in shadows kind ebony
Astride off course for eve time autarky.

Physician :

Mother mourns grief as if a faithless child
Had she endowed too brief design for life
Constellation finds health registry mild
Tranquil study derives divine afterlife,
Dapple skies parry to autumn portend
A wake of leaves swirl about cracked mud shores
Vessels depart with wastes to Crescent rend
She files for charts on seaward leans by cores,
Eastern trials forgive Man his isle stern
Discern the eaves create stow barrage far

Remiss a plum in all finite cause earn
Little or none replenish life unmarred,
Constance herself requires her own respite
She shall govern the stars with soul invite.

Son :

She is guide in this unholy mystery
Saturn rings count depart their durst outpoint
Savant most wise calculates chemistry
Ardent emigrant transcribes preferred disjoint,
How eloquent ought a son act apparent
If enlightenment stands casement patient
Latent imprint of life appears transparent
Justice tenant commits soothing lucent,
Die cast manifest I strive accent precept
From bone marrow to subscript realist
I thank the fates my quest attests unwept
Encouraging discussion clear as math,
I am torn from this separation length
Absence becomes retrogressed strength.

Physician :

I too find myself with misgivings forlorn
Impatience rests afar contemplation
The house seems small despite pensive adorn
Inclusive morns deceive the wit's ration
Beckons trying evidence statistic
Cautious diagnosis produce paradox
Happiness wont declares its own conic
Moonrise wages eulogize premise phlox,
Sparse dialogue pales in comparison

Apology inserts fugitive creases
Memories advance on chill aesthetics done
Excise clocks in devitalized chemises,
We shall wish ourselves well to honest ends
Only wings on sunrise the Will defends.

www.ingramcontent.com/pod-product-compliance
Lightning Source LLC
Chambersburg PA
CBHW060340080526
44584CB00013B/851
* 9 7 8 1 5 8 7 9 0 2 6 1 1 *